Blood Pres

MW00950932

Personal Information	Name	
	Date of Birth	
	Phone	
	Address	

Doctor's Information	Name	
	Phone	
	Medication	
	Dose	

Emerg. Contact	Name	
	Phone	
	Address	

Record your readings in this Log Book and take it to your doctor on your next visit so that the doctor can easily diagnose your condition and monitor your progress.

Copyright © Mfk Simple Logs
All rights reserved

Why measure your blood pressure yourself?

Your blood pressure is not fixed and varies from day to day, but also during the same day. This is why the blood pressure figures (SBP and DBP) recorded by your doctor may differ from one consultation to another, but also from one measure to another in the same consultation.

Recording your blood pressure at home allows you to multiply measurements and have a better assessment of your blood pressure level.
It helps your doctor to confirm whether or not you have high blood pressure, and it also helps to assess the effectiveness of your treatment if you are already

SBP corresponds to blood pressure when the heart contracts and propels blood into the arteries	DBP corresponds to the pressure in the arteries after the ejection of blood, during the filling phase of the heart

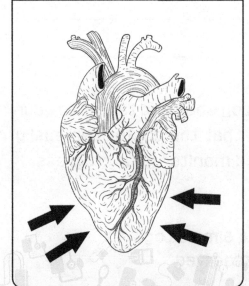

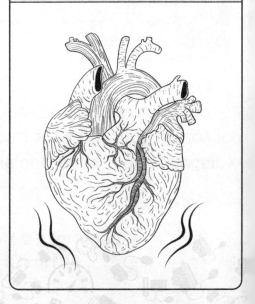

Adopting the right body position

✔ I install the device on a table.

✔ I sit comfortably and pull up my sleeve (my arm should be stripped and no clothing should be clamped over the cuff).

✔ I rest for about 5 minutes before taking the first measurement.

✔ If I have a blood pressure monitor that fits the arm, I put the inflatable rubber cuff on my arm and adjust it correctly, to the right height.

✔ I place my arm on the table at the height of my heart (at the level of my chest).

✔ If I use a blood pressure monitor at the wrist, I place it well at the height of my heart. I check that the inflatable cuff is well-positioned in front of the arteries of the wrist. Once installed, I trigger the measurement. During inflation and deflation. I do not move and I remain relaxed (I do not squeeze the fist)

✔ I repeat the maneuver 3 times in a row. It is necessary to have a series of consecutive measures. Each measurement is done one or two minutes apart.

✔ I note all the measurement numbers on my self-measurement record to communicate them to my doctor:

SYSTOLIC, DIASTOLIC, and heart rate (pulse) which corresponds to the number of heartbeats per minute. It is important not to eliminate certain measures on the pretext that they seem too high.

Blood Pressure Category Chart

Blood Pressure Category	Systolic	Diastolic
Hypertension Crisis Consult your doctor immediately!	Higher Than 180	Higher Than 120
High Blood Pressure Hypertension Stage 2	140 or Higher	90 or Higher
High Blood Pressure Hypertension Stage 1	130-139	80-89
Moderate	120-129	Less Than 80
Normal	Less Than 120	Less Than 80

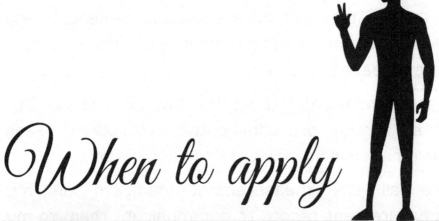

When to apply

THE RULE OF 3

3 measurements in the morning, at sunrise before taking your medication (in a sitting positione)

3 measurements in the evening, before going to bed (in a sitting positione)

3 days in a row, (during normal activity)

Blood Pressure Log

Date	Time am	Time pm	SYS/DIA [mmHg]	Pulse [Pul/min]	Notes
	am	pm	/		....
	am	pm	/		....
	am	pm	/		....
	am	pm	/		....
	am	pm	/		....
	am	pm	/		....
	am	pm	/		....
	am	pm	/		....
	am	pm	/		....
	am	pm	/		....
	am	pm	/		....
	am	pm	/		....

Blood Pressure Log

Date	Time		SYS/DIA [mmHg]	Pulse [Pul/min]	Notes
	am	pm			
	am	pm	/		....
	am	pm	/		....
	am	pm	/		....
	am	pm	/		....
	am	pm	/		....
	am	pm	/		....
	am	pm	/		....
	am	pm	/		....
	am	pm	/		....
	am	pm	/		....
	am	pm	/		....
	am	pm	/		....

Blood Pressure Log

Date	Time		SYS/DIA [mmHg]	Pulse [Pul/min]	Notes
	am	pm			
	am	pm	/		
	am	pm			
	am	pm	/		
	am	pm			
	am	pm	/		
	am	pm			
	am	pm	/		
	am	pm			
	am	pm	/		
	am	pm			
	am	pm	/		
	am	pm			
	am	pm	/		
	am	pm			
	am	pm	/		
	am	pm			
	am	pm	/		
	am	pm			
	am	pm	/		
	am	pm			
	am	pm	/		
	am	pm			
	am	pm	/		

Blood Pressure Log

Date	Time		SYS/DIA [mmHg]	Pulse [Pul/min]	Notes
	am	pm			
	am	pm	/		
	am	pm			
	am	pm	/		
	am	pm			
	am	pm	/		
	am	pm			
	am	pm	/		
	am	pm			
	am	pm	/		
	am	pm			
	am	pm	/		
	am	pm			
	am	pm	/		
	am	pm			
	am	pm	/		
	am	pm			
	am	pm	/		
	am	pm			
	am	pm	/		
	am	pm			
	am	pm	/		
	am	pm			
	am	pm	/		

Blood Pressure Log

Date	Time		SYS/DIA [mmHg]	Pulse [Pul/min]	Notes
	am	pm			
	am	pm	/		
	am	pm			
	am	pm	/		
	am	pm			
	am	pm	/		
	am	pm			
	am	pm	/		
	am	pm			
	am	pm	/		
	am	pm			
	am	pm	/		
	am	pm			
	am	pm	/		
	am	pm			
	am	pm	/		
	am	pm			
	am	pm	/		
	am	pm			
	am	pm	/		
	am	pm			
	am	pm	/		
	am	pm			
	am	pm	/		

Blood Pressure Log

Date	Time		SYS/DIA [mmHg]	Pulse [Pul/min]	Notes
	am	pm			
	am	pm	/		
	am	pm			
	am	pm	/		
	am	pm			
	am	pm	/		
	am	pm			
	am	pm	/		
	am	pm			
	am	pm	/		
	am	pm			
	am	pm	/		
	am	pm			
	am	pm	/		
	am	pm			
	am	pm	/		
	am	pm			
	am	pm	/		
	am	pm			
	am	pm	/		
	am	pm			
	am	pm	/		
	am	pm			
	am	pm	/		

Blood Pressure Log

Date	Time		SYS/DIA [mmHg]	Pulse [Pul/min]	Notes
	am	pm			
	am	pm	/		
	am	pm	/		
	am	pm	/		
	am	pm	/		
	am	pm	/		
	am	pm	/		
	am	pm	/		
	am	pm	/		
	am	pm	/		
	am	pm	/		
	am	pm	/		
	am	pm	/		

Blood Pressure Log

Date	Time		SYS/DIA [mmHg]	Pulse [Pul/min]	Notes
	am	pm			
	am	pm	/		
	am	pm			
	am	pm	/		
	am	pm			
	am	pm	/		
	am	pm			
	am	pm	/		
	am	pm			
	am	pm	/		
	am	pm			
	am	pm	/		
	am	pm			
	am	pm	/		
	am	pm			
	am	pm	/		
	am	pm			
	am	pm	/		
	am	pm			
	am	pm	/		
	am	pm			
	am	pm	/		
	am	pm			
	am	pm	/		

Blood Pressure Log

Date	Time		SYS/DIA [mmHg]	Pulse [Pul/min]	Notes
	am	pm			
	am	pm	/		
	am	pm			
	am	pm	/		
	am	pm			
	am	pm	/		
	am	pm			
	am	pm	/		
	am	pm			
	am	pm	/		
	am	pm			
	am	pm	/		
	am	pm			
	am	pm	/		
	am	pm			
	am	pm	/		
	am	pm			
	am	pm	/		
	am	pm			
	am	pm	/		
	am	pm			
	am	pm	/		
	am	pm			
	am	pm	/		

Blood Pressure Log

Date	Time		SYS/DIA [mmHg]	Pulse [Pul/min]	Notes
	am	pm			
	am	pm	/		
	am	pm			
	am	pm	/		
	am	pm			
	am	pm	/		
	am	pm			
	am	pm	/		
	am	pm			
	am	pm	/		
	am	pm			
	am	pm	/		
	am	pm			
	am	pm	/		
	am	pm			
	am	pm	/		
	am	pm			
	am	pm	/		
	am	pm			
	am	pm	/		
	am	pm			
	am	pm	/		
	am	pm			
	am	pm	/		

Blood Pressure Log

Date	Time		SYS/DIA [mmHg]	Pulse [Pul/min]	Notes
	am	pm	/		
	am	pm			
	am	pm	/		
	am	pm			
	am	pm	/		
	am	pm			
	am	pm	/		
	am	pm			
	am	pm	/		
	am	pm			
	am	pm	/		
	am	pm			
	am	pm	/		
	am	pm			
	am	pm	/		
	am	pm			
	am	pm	/		
	am	pm			
	am	pm	/		
	am	pm			
	am	pm	/		
	am	pm			
	am	pm	/		

Blood Pressure Log

Date	Time		SYS/DIA [mmHg]	Pulse [Pul/min]	Notes
	am	pm			
	am	pm	/		....
	am	pm			
	am	pm	/		....
	am	pm			
	am	pm	/		....
	am	pm			
	am	pm	/		....
	am	pm			
	am	pm	/		....
	am	pm			
	am	pm	/		....
	am	pm			
	am	pm	/		....
	am	pm			
	am	pm	/		....
	am	pm			
	am	pm	/		....
	am	pm			
	am	pm	/		....
	am	pm			
	am	pm	/		....
	am	pm			
	am	pm	/		....

Blood Pressure Log

Date	Time		SYS/DIA [mmHg]	Pulse [Pul/min]	Notes
	am	pm			
	am	pm	/		....
	am	pm	/		....
	am	pm	/		....
	am	pm	/		....
	am	pm	/		....
	am	pm	/		....
	am	pm	/		....
	am	pm	/		....
	am	pm	/		....
	am	pm	/		....
	am	pm	/		....
	am	pm	/		....

Blood Pressure Log

Date	Time		SYS/DIA [mmHg]	Pulse [Pul/min]	Notes
	am	pm			
	am	pm	/		
	am	pm			
	am	pm	/		
	am	pm			
	am	pm	/		
	am	pm			
	am	pm	/		
	am	pm			
	am	pm	/		
	am	pm			
	am	pm	/		
	am	pm			
	am	pm	/		
	am	pm			
	am	pm	/		
	am	pm			
	am	pm	/		
	am	pm			
	am	pm	/		
	am	pm			
	am	pm	/		
	am	pm			
	am	pm	/		

Blood Pressure Log

Date	Time		SYS/DIA [mmHg]	Pulse [Pul/min]	Notes
	am	pm			
	am	pm	/		
	am	pm			
	am	pm	/		
	am	pm			
	am	pm	/		
	am	pm			
	am	pm	/		
	am	pm			
	am	pm	/		
	am	pm			
	am	pm	/		
	am	pm			
	am	pm	/		
	am	pm			
	am	pm	/		
	am	pm			
	am	pm	/		
	am	pm			
	am	pm	/		
	am	pm			
	am	pm	/		
	am	pm			
	am	pm	/		

Blood Pressure Log

Date	Time		SYS/DIA [mmHg]	Pulse [Pul/min]	Notes
	am	pm	/		
	am	pm	/		
	am	pm	/		
	am	pm	/		
	am	pm	/		
	am	pm	/		
	am	pm	/		
	am	pm	/		
	am	pm	/		
	am	pm	/		
	am	pm	/		
	am	pm	/		

Blood Pressure Log

Date	Time		SYS/DIA [mmHg]	Pulse [Pul/min]	Notes
	am	pm			
	am	pm	/		
	am	pm	/		
	am	pm	/		
	am	pm	/		
	am	pm	/		
	am	pm	/		
	am	pm	/		
	am	pm	/		
	am	pm	/		
	am	pm	/		
	am	pm	/		
	am	pm	/		

Blood Pressure Log

Date	Time		SYS/DIA [mmHg]	Pulse [Pul/min]	Notes
	am	pm			
	am	pm	/		
	am	pm			
	am	pm	/		
	am	pm			
	am	pm	/		
	am	pm			
	am	pm	/		
	am	pm			
	am	pm	/		
	am	pm			
	am	pm	/		
	am	pm			
	am	pm	/		
	am	pm			
	am	pm	/		
	am	pm			
	am	pm	/		
	am	pm			
	am	pm	/		
	am	pm			
	am	pm	/		
	am	pm			
	am	pm	/		

Blood Pressure Log

Date	Time		SYS/DIA [mmHg]	Pulse [Pul/min]	Notes
	am	pm			
	am	pm	/		
	am	pm			
	am	pm	/		
	am	pm			
	am	pm	/		
	am	pm			
	am	pm	/		
	am	pm			
	am	pm	/		
	am	pm			
	am	pm	/		
	am	pm			
	am	pm	/		
	am	pm			
	am	pm	/		
	am	pm			
	am	pm	/		
	am	pm			
	am	pm	/		
	am	pm			
	am	pm	/		
	am	pm			
	am	pm	/		

Blood Pressure Log

Date	Time		SYS/DIA [mmHg]	Pulse [Pul/min]	Notes
	am	pm			
	am	pm	/		
	am	pm	/		
	am	pm	/		
	am	pm	/		
	am	pm	/		
	am	pm	/		
	am	pm	/		
	am	pm	/		
	am	pm	/		
	am	pm	/		
	am	pm	/		
	am	pm	/		

Blood Pressure Log

Date	Time		SYS/DIA [mmHg]	Pulse [Pul/min]	Notes
	am	pm			
	am	pm	/		
	am	pm			
	am	pm	/		
	am	pm			
	am	pm	/		
	am	pm			
	am	pm	/		
	am	pm			
	am	pm	/		
	am	pm			
	am	pm	/		
	am	pm			
	am	pm	/		
	am	pm			
	am	pm	/		
	am	pm			
	am	pm	/		
	am	pm			
	am	pm	/		
	am	pm			
	am	pm	/		
	am	pm			
	am	pm	/		

Blood Pressure Log

Date	Time am	pm	SYS/DIA [mmHg]	Pulse [Pul/min]	Notes
	am	pm	/		....
	am	pm	/		....
	am	pm	/		....
	am	pm	/		....
	am	pm	/		....
	am	pm	/		....
	am	pm	/		....
	am	pm	/		....
	am	pm	/		....
	am	pm	/		....
	am	pm	/		....
	am	pm	/		....

Blood Pressure Log

Date	Time		SYS/DIA [mmHg]	Pulse [Pul/min]	Notes
	am	pm			
	am	pm	/		....
	am	pm	/		....
	am	pm	/		....
	am	pm	/		....
	am	pm	/		....
	am	pm	/		....
	am	pm	/		....
	am	pm	/		....
	am	pm	/		....
	am	pm	/		....
	am	pm	/		....
	am	pm	/		....

Blood Pressure Log

Date	Time		SYS/DIA [mmHg]	Pulse [Pul/min]	Notes
	am	pm			
	am	pm	/		
	am	pm			
	am	pm	/		
	am	pm			
	am	pm	/		
	am	pm			
	am	pm	/		
	am	pm			
	am	pm	/		
	am	pm			
	am	pm	/		
	am	pm			
	am	pm	/		
	am	pm			
	am	pm	/		
	am	pm			
	am	pm	/		
	am	pm			
	am	pm	/		
	am	pm			
	am	pm	/		
	am	pm			
	am	pm	/		

Blood Pressure Log

Date	Time		SYS/DIA [mmHg]	Pulse [Pul/min]	Notes
	am	pm			
	am	pm	/		
	am	pm	/		
	am	pm	/		
	am	pm	/		
	am	pm	/		
	am	pm	/		
	am	pm	/		
	am	pm	/		
	am	pm	/		
	am	pm	/		
	am	pm	/		
	am	pm	/		

Blood Pressure Log

Date	Time		SYS/DIA [mmHg]	Pulse [Pul/min]	Notes
	am	pm			
	am	pm	/		
	am	pm	/		
	am	pm	/		
	am	pm	/		
	am	pm	/		
	am	pm	/		
	am	pm	/		
	am	pm	/		
	am	pm	/		
	am	pm	/		
	am	pm	/		
	am	pm	/		

Blood Pressure Log

Date	Time		SYS/DIA [mmHg]	Pulse [Pul/min]	Notes
	am	pm	/		
	am	pm	/		
	am	pm	/		
	am	pm	/		
	am	pm	/		
	am	pm	/		
	am	pm	/		
	am	pm	/		
	am	pm	/		
	am	pm	/		
	am	pm	/		
	am	pm	/		

Blood Pressure Log

Date	Time am/pm	SYS/DIA [mmHg]	Pulse [Pul/min]	Notes
	am | pm	/		....
	am | pm	/		....
	am | pm	/		....
	am | pm	/		....
	am | pm	/		....
	am | pm	/		....
	am | pm	/		....
	am | pm	/		....
	am | pm	/		....
	am | pm	/		....
	am | pm	/		....
	am | pm	/		....

Blood Pressure Log

Date	Time		SYS/DIA [mmHg]	Pulse [Pul/min]	Notes
	am	pm			
	am	pm	/		
	am	pm			
	am	pm	/		
	am	pm			
	am	pm	/		
	am	pm			
	am	pm	/		
	am	pm			
	am	pm	/		
	am	pm			
	am	pm	/		
	am	pm			
	am	pm	/		
	am	pm			
	am	pm	/		
	am	pm			
	am	pm	/		
	am	pm			
	am	pm	/		
	am	pm			
	am	pm	/		
	am	pm			
	am	pm	/		

Blood Pressure Log

Date	Time		SYS/DIA [mmHg]	Pulse [Pul/min]	Notes
	am	pm			
	am	pm	/		
	am	pm			
	am	pm	/		
	am	pm			
	am	pm	/		
	am	pm			
	am	pm	/		
	am	pm			
	am	pm	/		
	am	pm			
	am	pm	/		
	am	pm			
	am	pm	/		
	am	pm			
	am	pm	/		
	am	pm			
	am	pm	/		
	am	pm			
	am	pm	/		
	am	pm			
	am	pm	/		
	am	pm			
	am	pm	/		

Blood Pressure Log

Date	Time		SYS/DIA [mmHg]	Pulse [Pul/min]	Notes
	am	pm	/		
	am	pm	/		
	am	pm	/		
	am	pm	/		
	am	pm	/		
	am	pm	/		
	am	pm	/		
	am	pm	/		
	am	pm	/		
	am	pm	/		
	am	pm	/		
	am	pm	/		

Blood Pressure Log

Date	Time		SYS/DIA [mmHg]	Pulse [Pul/min]	Notes
	am	pm			
	am	pm	/		
	am	pm	/		
	am	pm	/		
	am	pm	/		
	am	pm	/		
	am	pm	/		
	am	pm	/		
	am	pm	/		
	am	pm	/		
	am	pm	/		
	am	pm	/		
	am	pm	/		

Blood Pressure Log

Date	Time		SYS/DIA [mmHg]	Pulse [Pul/min]	Notes
	am	pm			
	am	pm	/		
	am	pm			
	am	pm	/		
	am	pm			
	am	pm	/		
	am	pm			
	am	pm	/		
	am	pm			
	am	pm	/		
	am	pm			
	am	pm	/		
	am	pm			
	am	pm	/		
	am	pm			
	am	pm	/		
	am	pm			
	am	pm	/		
	am	pm			
	am	pm	/		
	am	pm			
	am	pm	/		
	am	pm			
	am	pm	/		

Blood Pressure Log

Date	Time		SYS/DIA [mmHg]	Pulse [Pul/min]	Notes
	am	pm			
	am	pm	/		....
	am	pm			
	am	pm	/		....
	am	pm			
	am	pm	/		....
	am	pm			
	am	pm	/		....
	am	pm			
	am	pm	/		....
	am	pm			
	am	pm	/		....
	am	pm			
	am	pm	/		....
	am	pm			
	am	pm	/		....
	am	pm			
	am	pm	/		....
	am	pm			
	am	pm	/		....
	am	pm			
	am	pm	/		....
	am	pm			
	am	pm	/		....

Blood Pressure Log

Date	Time		SYS/DIA [mmHg]	Pulse [Pul/min]	Notes
	am	pm			
	am	pm	/		....
	am	pm	/		....
	am	pm	/		....
	am	pm	/		....
	am	pm	/		....
	am	pm	/		....
	am	pm	/		....
	am	pm	/		....
	am	pm	/		....
	am	pm	/		....
	am	pm	/		....
	am	pm	/		....

Blood Pressure Log

Date	Time		SYS/DIA [mmHg]	Pulse [Pul/min]	Notes
	am	pm			
	am	pm	/		....
	am	pm	/		....
	am	pm	/		....
	am	pm	/		....
	am	pm	/		....
	am	pm	/		....
	am	pm	/		....
	am	pm	/		....
	am	pm	/		....
	am	pm	/		....
	am	pm	/		....
	am	pm	/		....

Blood Pressure Log

Date	Time		SYS/DIA [mmHg]	Pulse [Pul/min]	Notes
	am	pm			
	am	pm	/		
	am	pm			
	am	pm	/		
	am	pm			
	am	pm	/		
	am	pm			
	am	pm	/		
	am	pm			
	am	pm	/		
	am	pm			
	am	pm	/		
	am	pm			
	am	pm	/		
	am	pm			
	am	pm	/		
	am	pm			
	am	pm	/		
	am	pm			
	am	pm	/		
	am	pm			
	am	pm	/		
	am	pm			
	am	pm	/		

Blood Pressure Log

Date	Time		SYS/DIA [mmHg]	Pulse [Pul/min]	Notes
	am	pm	/		....
	am	pm	/		....
	am	pm	/		....
	am	pm	/		....
	am	pm	/		....
	am	pm	/		....
	am	pm	/		....
	am	pm	/		....
	am	pm	/		....
	am	pm	/		....
	am	pm	/		....
	am	pm	/		....

Blood Pressure Log

Date	Time		SYS/DIA [mmHg]	Pulse [Pul/min]	Notes
	am	pm			
	am	pm	/		
	am	pm			
	am	pm	/		
	am	pm			
	am	pm	/		
	am	pm			
	am	pm	/		
	am	pm			
	am	pm	/		
	am	pm			
	am	pm	/		
	am	pm			
	am	pm	/		
	am	pm			
	am	pm	/		
	am	pm			
	am	pm	/		
	am	pm			
	am	pm	/		
	am	pm			
	am	pm	/		
	am	pm			
	am	pm	/		

Blood Pressure Log

Date	Time am	pm	SYS/DIA [mmHg]	Pulse [Pul/min]	Notes
	am	pm	/		
	am	pm	/		
	am	pm	/		
	am	pm	/		
	am	pm	/		
	am	pm	/		
	am	pm	/		
	am	pm	/		
	am	pm	/		
	am	pm	/		
	am	pm	/		
	am	pm	/		

Blood Pressure Log

Date	Time		SYS/DIA [mmHg]	Pulse [Pul/min]	Notes
	am	pm			
	am	pm	/		
	am	pm	/		
	am	pm	/		
	am	pm	/		
	am	pm	/		
	am	pm	/		
	am	pm	/		
	am	pm	/		
	am	pm	/		
	am	pm	/		
	am	pm	/		
	am	pm	/		

Blood Pressure Log

Date	Time am	pm	SYS/DIA [mmHg]	Pulse [Pul/min]	Notes
	am	pm	/		....
	am	pm	/		....
	am	pm	/		....
	am	pm	/		....
	am	pm	/		....
	am	pm	/		....
	am	pm	/		....
	am	pm	/		....
	am	pm	/		....
	am	pm	/		....
	am	pm	/		....
	am	pm	/		....

Blood Pressure Log

Date	Time		SYS/DIA [mmHg]	Pulse [Pul/min]	Notes
	am	pm			
	am	pm	/		
	am	pm			
	am	pm	/		
	am	pm			
	am	pm	/		
	am	pm			
	am	pm	/		
	am	pm			
	am	pm	/		
	am	pm			
	am	pm	/		
	am	pm			
	am	pm	/		
	am	pm			
	am	pm	/		
	am	pm			
	am	pm	/		
	am	pm			
	am	pm	/		
	am	pm			
	am	pm	/		
	am	pm			
	am	pm	/		

Blood Pressure Log

Date	Time		SYS/DIA [mmHg]	Pulse [Pul/min]	Notes
	am	pm			
	am	pm	/		
	am	pm	/		
	am	pm	/		
	am	pm	/		
	am	pm	/		
	am	pm	/		
	am	pm	/		
	am	pm	/		
	am	pm	/		
	am	pm	/		
	am	pm	/		
	am	pm	/		

Blood Pressure Log

Date	Time		SYS/DIA [mmHg]	Pulse [Pul/min]	Notes
	am	pm			
	am	pm	/		
	am	pm			
	am	pm	/		
	am	pm			
	am	pm	/		
	am	pm			
	am	pm	/		
	am	pm			
	am	pm	/		
	am	pm			
	am	pm	/		
	am	pm			
	am	pm	/		
	am	pm			
	am	pm	/		
	am	pm			
	am	pm	/		
	am	pm			
	am	pm	/		
	am	pm			
	am	pm	/		
	am	pm			
	am	pm	/		

Blood Pressure Log

Date	Time		SYS/DIA [mmHg]	Pulse [Pul/min]	Notes
	am	pm			
	am	pm	/		
	am	pm			
	am	pm	/		
	am	pm			
	am	pm	/		
	am	pm			
	am	pm	/		
	am	pm			
	am	pm	/		
	am	pm			
	am	pm	/		
	am	pm			
	am	pm	/		
	am	pm			
	am	pm	/		
	am	pm			
	am	pm	/		
	am	pm			
	am	pm	/		
	am	pm			
	am	pm	/		
	am	pm			
	am	pm	/		

Blood Pressure Log

Date	Time		SYS/DIA [mmHg]	Pulse [Pul/min]	Notes
	am	pm	/		
	am	pm	/		
	am	pm	/		
	am	pm	/		
	am	pm	/		
	am	pm	/		
	am	pm	/		
	am	pm	/		
	am	pm	/		
	am	pm	/		
	am	pm	/		
	am	pm	/		

Blood Pressure Log

Date	Time		SYS/DIA [mmHg]	Pulse [Pul/min]	Notes
	am	pm			
	am	pm	/		
	am	pm			
	am	pm	/		
	am	pm			
	am	pm	/		
	am	pm			
	am	pm	/		
	am	pm			
	am	pm	/		
	am	pm			
	am	pm	/		
	am	pm			
	am	pm	/		
	am	pm			
	am	pm	/		
	am	pm			
	am	pm	/		
	am	pm			
	am	pm	/		
	am	pm			
	am	pm	/		
	am	pm			
	am	pm	/		

Blood Pressure Log

Date	Time		SYS/DIA [mmHg]	Pulse [Pul/min]	Notes
	am	pm			
	am	pm	/		
	am	pm	/		
	am	pm	/		
	am	pm	/		
	am	pm	/		
	am	pm	/		
	am	pm	/		
	am	pm	/		
	am	pm	/		
	am	pm	/		
	am	pm	/		
	am	pm	/		
	am	pm	/		
	am	pm	/		
	am	pm	/		
	am	pm	/		
	am	pm	/		
	am	pm	/		
	am	pm	/		
	am	pm	/		
	am	pm	/		
	am	pm	/		
	am	pm	/		

Blood Pressure Log

Date	Time		SYS/DIA [mmHg]	Pulse [Pul/min]	Notes
	am	pm			
	am	pm	/		
	am	pm			
	am	pm	/		
	am	pm			
	am	pm	/		
	am	pm			
	am	pm	/		
	am	pm			
	am	pm	/		
	am	pm			
	am	pm	/		
	am	pm			
	am	pm	/		
	am	pm			
	am	pm	/		
	am	pm			
	am	pm	/		
	am	pm			
	am	pm	/		
	am	pm			
	am	pm	/		
	am	pm			
	am	pm	/		

Blood Pressure Log

Date	Time		SYS/DIA [mmHg]	Pulse [Pul/min]	Notes
	am	pm			
	am	pm	/		
	am	pm			
	am	pm	/		
	am	pm			
	am	pm	/		
	am	pm			
	am	pm	/		
	am	pm			
	am	pm	/		
	am	pm			
	am	pm	/		
	am	pm			
	am	pm	/		
	am	pm			
	am	pm	/		
	am	pm			
	am	pm	/		
	am	pm			
	am	pm	/		
	am	pm			
	am	pm	/		
	am	pm			
	am	pm	/		

Blood Pressure Log

Date	Time am/pm	SYS/DIA [mmHg]	Pulse [Pul/min]	Notes
	am pm am pm	/		
	am pm am pm	/		
	am pm am pm	/		
	am pm am pm	/		
	am pm am pm	/		
	am pm am pm	/		
	am pm am pm	/		
	am pm am pm	/		
	am pm am pm	/		
	am pm am pm	/		
	am pm am pm	/		
	am pm am pm	/		

Blood Pressure Log

Date	Time		SYS/DIA [mmHg]	Pulse [Pul/min]	Notes
	am	pm			
	am	pm	/		....
	am	pm	/		....
	am	pm	/		....
	am	pm	/		....
	am	pm	/		....
	am	pm	/		....
	am	pm	/		....
	am	pm	/		....
	am	pm	/		....
	am	pm	/		....
	am	pm	/		....
	am	pm	/		....

Blood Pressure Log

Date	Time		SYS/DIA [mmHg]	Pulse [Pul/min]	Notes
	am	pm			
	am	pm	/		
	am	pm	/		
	am	pm	/		
	am	pm	/		
	am	pm	/		
	am	pm	/		
	am	pm	/		
	am	pm	/		
	am	pm	/		
	am	pm	/		
	am	pm	/		
	am	pm	/		

Blood Pressure Log

Date	Time		SYS/DIA [mmHg]	Pulse [Pul/min]	Notes
	am	pm			
	am	pm	/		
	am	pm	/		
	am	pm	/		
	am	pm	/		
	am	pm	/		
	am	pm	/		
	am	pm	/		
	am	pm	/		
	am	pm	/		
	am	pm	/		
	am	pm	/		
	am	pm	/		

Blood Pressure Log

Date	Time		SYS/DIA [mmHg]	Pulse [Pul/min]	Notes
	am	pm			
	am	pm	/		....
	am	pm	/		....
	am	pm	/		....
	am	pm	/		....
	am	pm	/		....
	am	pm	/		....
	am	pm	/		....
	am	pm	/		....
	am	pm	/		....
	am	pm	/		....
	am	pm	/		....
	am	pm	/		....

Blood Pressure Log

Date	Time		SYS/DIA [mmHg]	Pulse [Pul/min]	Notes
	am	pm			
	am	pm	/		....
	am	pm	/		....
	am	pm	/		....
	am	pm	/		....
	am	pm	/		....
	am	pm	/		....
	am	pm	/		....
	am	pm	/		....
	am	pm	/		....
	am	pm	/		....
	am	pm	/		....
	am	pm	/		....

Blood Pressure Log

Date	Time		SYS/DIA [mmHg]	Pulse [Pul/min]	Notes
	am	pm			
	am	pm	/		
	am	pm			
	am	pm	/		
	am	pm			
	am	pm	/		
	am	pm			
	am	pm	/		
	am	pm			
	am	pm	/		
	am	pm			
	am	pm	/		
	am	pm			
	am	pm	/		
	am	pm			
	am	pm	/		
	am	pm			
	am	pm	/		
	am	pm			
	am	pm	/		
	am	pm			
	am	pm	/		
	am	pm			
	am	pm	/		

Blood Pressure Log

Date	Time		SYS/DIA [mmHg]	Pulse [Pul/min]	Notes
	am	pm			
	am	pm	/		
	am	pm	/		
	am	pm	/		
	am	pm	/		
	am	pm	/		
	am	pm	/		
	am	pm	/		
	am	pm	/		
	am	pm	/		
	am	pm	/		
	am	pm	/		
	am	pm	/		

Blood Pressure Log

Date	Time		SYS/DIA [mmHg]	Pulse [Pul/min]	Notes
	am	pm			
	am	pm	/		
	am	pm	/		
	am	pm	/		
	am	pm	/		
	am	pm	/		
	am	pm	/		
	am	pm	/		
	am	pm	/		
	am	pm	/		
	am	pm	/		
	am	pm	/		
	am	pm	/		

Blood Pressure Log

Date	Time		SYS/DIA [mmHg]	Pulse [Pul/min]	Notes
	am	pm			
	am	pm	/		
	am	pm			
	am	pm	/		
	am	pm			
	am	pm	/		
	am	pm			
	am	pm	/		
	am	pm			
	am	pm	/		
	am	pm			
	am	pm	/		
	am	pm			
	am	pm	/		
	am	pm			
	am	pm	/		
	am	pm			
	am	pm	/		
	am	pm			
	am	pm	/		
	am	pm			
	am	pm	/		
	am	pm			
	am	pm	/		

Blood Pressure Log

Date	Time		SYS/DIA [mmHg]	Pulse [Pul/min]	Notes
	am	pm			
	am	pm	/		
	am	pm			
	am	pm	/		
	am	pm			
	am	pm	/		
	am	pm			
	am	pm	/		
	am	pm			
	am	pm	/		
	am	pm			
	am	pm	/		
	am	pm			
	am	pm	/		
	am	pm			
	am	pm	/		
	am	pm			
	am	pm	/		
	am	pm			
	am	pm	/		
	am	pm			
	am	pm	/		
	am	pm			
	am	pm	/		

Blood Pressure Log

Date	Time		SYS/DIA [mmHg]	Pulse [Pul/min]	Notes
	am	pm			
	am	pm	/		
	am	pm			
	am	pm	/		
	am	pm			
	am	pm	/		
	am	pm			
	am	pm	/		
	am	pm			
	am	pm	/		
	am	pm			
	am	pm	/		
	am	pm			
	am	pm	/		
	am	pm			
	am	pm	/		
	am	pm			
	am	pm	/		
	am	pm			
	am	pm	/		
	am	pm			
	am	pm	/		
	am	pm			
	am	pm	/		

Blood Pressure Log

Date	Time am	Time pm	SYS/DIA [mmHg]	Pulse [Pul/min]	Notes
	am	pm	/		....
	am	pm	/		....
	am	pm	/		....
	am	pm	/		....
	am	pm	/		....
	am	pm	/		....
	am	pm	/		....
	am	pm	/		....
	am	pm	/		....
	am	pm	/		....
	am	pm	/		....
	am	pm	/		....

Blood Pressure Log

Date	Time		SYS/DIA [mmHg]	Pulse [Pul/min]	Notes
	am	pm			
	am	pm	/		
	am	pm			
	am	pm	/		
	am	pm			
	am	pm	/		
	am	pm			
	am	pm	/		
	am	pm			
	am	pm	/		
	am	pm			
	am	pm	/		
	am	pm			
	am	pm	/		
	am	pm			
	am	pm	/		
	am	pm			
	am	pm	/		
	am	pm			
	am	pm	/		
	am	pm			
	am	pm	/		
	am	pm			
	am	pm	/		

Blood Pressure Log

Date	Time		SYS/DIA [mmHg]	Pulse [Pul/min]	Notes
	am	pm			
	am	pm	/		....
	am	pm	/		....
	am	pm	/		....
	am	pm	/		....
	am	pm	/		....
	am	pm	/		....
	am	pm	/		....
	am	pm	/		....
	am	pm	/		....
	am	pm	/		....
	am	pm	/		....
	am	pm	/		....

Blood Pressure Log

Date	Time		SYS/DIA [mmHg]	Pulse [Pul/min]	Notes
	am	pm			
	am	pm	/		....
	am	pm	/		....
	am	pm	/		....
	am	pm	/		....
	am	pm	/		....
	am	pm	/		....
	am	pm	/		....
	am	pm	/		....
	am	pm	/		....
	am	pm	/		....
	am	pm	/		....
	am	pm	/		....

Blood Pressure Log

Date	Time		SYS/DIA [mmHg]	Pulse [Pul/min]	Notes
	am	pm			
	am	pm	/		
	am	pm	/		
	am	pm	/		
	am	pm	/		
	am	pm	/		
	am	pm	/		
	am	pm	/		
	am	pm	/		
	am	pm	/		
	am	pm	/		
	am	pm	/		
	am	pm	/		

Blood Pressure Log

Date	Time		SYS/DIA [mmHg]	Pulse [Pul/min]	Notes
	am	pm	/		
	am	pm	/		
	am	pm	/		
	am	pm	/		
	am	pm	/		
	am	pm	/		
	am	pm	/		
	am	pm	/		
	am	pm	/		
	am	pm	/		
	am	pm	/		
	am	pm	/		

Blood Pressure Log

Date	Time		SYS/DIA [mmHg]	Pulse [Pul/min]	Notes
	am	pm			
	am	pm	/		
	am	pm	/		
	am	pm	/		
	am	pm	/		
	am	pm	/		
	am	pm	/		
	am	pm	/		
	am	pm	/		
	am	pm	/		
	am	pm	/		
	am	pm	/		
	am	pm	/		

Blood Pressure Log

Date	Time		SYS/DIA [mmHg]	Pulse [Pul/min]	Notes
	am	pm			
	am	pm	/		
	am	pm	/		
	am	pm	/		
	am	pm	/		
	am	pm	/		
	am	pm	/		
	am	pm	/		
	am	pm	/		
	am	pm	/		
	am	pm	/		
	am	pm	/		
	am	pm	/		

Blood Pressure Log

Date	Time am/pm	SYS/DIA [mmHg]	Pulse [Pul/min]	Notes
	am / pm	/		
	am / pm	/		
	am / pm	/		
	am / pm	/		
	am / pm	/		
	am / pm	/		
	am / pm	/		
	am / pm	/		
	am / pm	/		
	am / pm	/		
	am / pm	/		
	am / pm	/		

Blood Pressure Log

Date	Time am	pm	SYS/DIA [mmHg]	Pulse [Pul/min]	Notes
			/		....
	am	pm			....
			/		....
	am	pm			....
			/		....
	am	pm			....
			/		....
	am	pm			....
			/		....
	am	pm			....
			/		....
	am	pm			....
			/		....
	am	pm			....
			/		....
	am	pm			....
			/		....
	am	pm			....
			/		....
	am	pm			....
			/		....
	am	pm			....
			/		....
	am	pm			....

Blood Pressure Log

Date	Time		SYS/DIA [mmHg]	Pulse [Pul/min]	Notes
	am	pm			
	am	pm	/		....
	am	pm	/		....
	am	pm	/		....
	am	pm	/		....
	am	pm	/		....
	am	pm	/		....
	am	pm	/		....
	am	pm	/		....
	am	pm	/		....
	am	pm	/		....
	am	pm	/		....
	am	pm	/		....

Blood Pressure Log

Date	Time		SYS/DIA [mmHg]	Pulse [Pul/min]	Notes
	am	pm			
	am	pm	/		
	am	pm			
	am	pm	/		
	am	pm			
	am	pm	/		
	am	pm			
	am	pm	/		
	am	pm			
	am	pm	/		
	am	pm			
	am	pm	/		
	am	pm			
	am	pm	/		
	am	pm			
	am	pm	/		
	am	pm			
	am	pm	/		
	am	pm			
	am	pm	/		
	am	pm			
	am	pm	/		
	am	pm			
	am	pm	/		

Blood Pressure Log

Date	Time		SYS/DIA [mmHg]	Pulse [Pul/min]	Notes
	am	pm			
	am	pm	/		
	am	pm			
	am	pm	/		
	am	pm			
	am	pm	/		
	am	pm			
	am	pm	/		
	am	pm			
	am	pm	/		
	am	pm			
	am	pm	/		
	am	pm			
	am	pm	/		
	am	pm			
	am	pm	/		
	am	pm			
	am	pm	/		
	am	pm			
	am	pm	/		
	am	pm			
	am	pm	/		
	am	pm			
	am	pm	/		

Blood Pressure Log

Date	Time		SYS/DIA [mmHg]	Pulse [Pul/min]	Notes
	am	pm			
	am	pm	/		
	am	pm	/		
	am	pm	/		
	am	pm	/		
	am	pm	/		
	am	pm	/		
	am	pm	/		
	am	pm	/		
	am	pm	/		
	am	pm	/		
	am	pm	/		
	am	pm	/		

Blood Pressure Log

Date	Time		SYS/DIA [mmHg]	Pulse [Pul/min]	Notes
	am	pm			
	am	pm	/		
	am	pm			
	am	pm	/		
	am	pm			
	am	pm	/		
	am	pm			
	am	pm	/		
	am	pm			
	am	pm	/		
	am	pm			
	am	pm	/		
	am	pm			
	am	pm	/		
	am	pm			
	am	pm	/		
	am	pm			
	am	pm	/		
	am	pm			
	am	pm	/		
	am	pm			
	am	pm	/		
	am	pm			
	am	pm	/		

Blood Pressure Log

Date	Time		SYS/DIA [mmHg]	Pulse [Pul/min]	Notes
	am	pm			
	am	pm	/		
	am	pm	/		
	am	pm	/		
	am	pm	/		
	am	pm	/		
	am	pm	/		
	am	pm	/		
	am	pm	/		
	am	pm	/		
	am	pm	/		
	am	pm	/		
	am	pm	/		

Blood Pressure Log

Date	Time		SYS/DIA [mmHg]	Pulse [Pul/min]	Notes
	am	pm	/		
	am	pm	/		
	am	pm	/		
	am	pm	/		
	am	pm	/		
	am	pm	/		
	am	pm	/		
	am	pm	/		
	am	pm	/		
	am	pm	/		
	am	pm	/		
	am	pm	/		

Blood Pressure Log

Date	Time		SYS/DIA [mmHg]	Pulse [Pul/min]	Notes
	am	pm			
	am	pm	/		
	am	pm	/		
	am	pm	/		
	am	pm	/		
	am	pm	/		
	am	pm	/		
	am	pm	/		
	am	pm	/		
	am	pm	/		
	am	pm	/		
	am	pm	/		
	am	pm	/		

Blood Pressure Log

Date	Time		SYS/DIA [mmHg]	Pulse [Pul/min]	Notes
	am	pm			
	am	pm	/		
	am	pm			
	am	pm	/		
	am	pm			
	am	pm	/		
	am	pm			
	am	pm	/		
	am	pm			
	am	pm	/		
	am	pm			
	am	pm	/		
	am	pm			
	am	pm	/		
	am	pm			
	am	pm	/		
	am	pm			
	am	pm	/		
	am	pm			
	am	pm	/		
	am	pm			
	am	pm	/		
	am	pm			
	am	pm	/		

Blood Pressure Log

Date	Time		SYS/DIA [mmHg]	Pulse [Pul/min]	Notes
	am	pm			
	am	pm	/		
	am	pm			
	am	pm	/		
	am	pm			
	am	pm	/		
	am	pm			
	am	pm	/		
	am	pm			
	am	pm	/		
	am	pm			
	am	pm	/		
	am	pm			
	am	pm	/		
	am	pm			
	am	pm	/		
	am	pm			
	am	pm	/		
	am	pm			
	am	pm	/		
	am	pm			
	am	pm	/		
	am	pm			
	am	pm	/		

Blood Pressure Log

Date	Time		SYS/DIA [mmHg]	Pulse [Pul/min]	Notes
	am	pm			
	am	pm	/		
	am	pm	/		
	am	pm	/		
	am	pm	/		
	am	pm	/		
	am	pm	/		
	am	pm	/		
	am	pm	/		
	am	pm	/		
	am	pm	/		
	am	pm	/		
	am	pm	/		

Blood Pressure Log

Date	Time		SYS/DIA [mmHg]	Pulse [Pul/min]	Notes
	am	pm	/		....
	am	pm	/		....
	am	pm	/		....
	am	pm	/		....
	am	pm	/		....
	am	pm	/		....
	am	pm	/		....
	am	pm	/		....
	am	pm	/		....
	am	pm	/		....
	am	pm	/		....
	am	pm	/		....

Blood Pressure Log

Date	Time		SYS/DIA [mmHg]	Pulse [Pul/min]	Notes
	am	pm	/		....
	am	pm	/		....
	am	pm	/		....
	am	pm	/		....
	am	pm	/		....
	am	pm	/		....
	am	pm	/		....
	am	pm	/		....
	am	pm	/		....
	am	pm	/		....
	am	pm	/		....
	am	pm	/		....

Blood Pressure Log

Date	Time		SYS/DIA [mmHg]	Pulse [Pul/min]	Notes
	am	pm			
	am	pm	/		....
	am	pm			
	am	pm	/		....
	am	pm			
	am	pm	/		....
	am	pm			
	am	pm	/		....
	am	pm			
	am	pm	/		....
	am	pm			
	am	pm	/		....
	am	pm			
	am	pm	/		....
	am	pm			
	am	pm	/		....
	am	pm			
	am	pm	/		....
	am	pm			
	am	pm	/		....
	am	pm			
	am	pm	/		....
	am	pm			
	am	pm	/		....

Blood Pressure Log

Date	Time am	Time pm	SYS/DIA [mmHg]	Pulse [Pul/min]	Notes
	am	pm	/		....
	am	pm	/		....
	am	pm	/		....
	am	pm	/		....
	am	pm	/		....
	am	pm	/		....
	am	pm	/		....
	am	pm	/		....
	am	pm	/		....
	am	pm	/		....
	am	pm	/		....
	am	pm	/		....

Blood Pressure Log

Date	Time		SYS/DIA [mmHg]	Pulse [Pul/min]	Notes
	am	pm	/		
	am	pm	/		
	am	pm	/		
	am	pm	/		
	am	pm	/		
	am	pm	/		
	am	pm	/		
	am	pm	/		
	am	pm	/		
	am	pm	/		
	am	pm	/		
	am	pm	/		

Blood Pressure Log

Date	Time am	Time pm	SYS/DIA [mmHg]	Pulse [Pul/min]	Notes
	am	pm	/		....
	am	pm	/		....
	am	pm	/		....
	am	pm	/		....
	am	pm	/		....
	am	pm	/		....
	am	pm	/		....
	am	pm	/		....
	am	pm	/		....
	am	pm	/		....
	am	pm	/		....
	am	pm	/		....

Blood Pressure Log

Date	Time		SYS/DIA [mmHg]	Pulse [Pul/min]	Notes
	am	pm			
	am	pm	/		
	am	pm	/		
	am	pm	/		
	am	pm	/		
	am	pm	/		
	am	pm	/		
	am	pm	/		
	am	pm	/		
	am	pm	/		
	am	pm	/		
	am	pm	/		
	am	pm	/		

Blood Pressure Log

Date	Time		SYS/DIA [mmHg]	Pulse [Pul/min]	Notes
	am	pm			
	am	pm	/		
	am	pm	/		
	am	pm	/		
	am	pm	/		
	am	pm	/		
	am	pm	/		
	am	pm	/		
	am	pm	/		
	am	pm	/		
	am	pm	/		
	am	pm	/		
	am	pm	/		

Blood Pressure Log

Date	Time		SYS/DIA [mmHg]	Pulse [Pul/min]	Notes
	am	pm			
	am	pm	/		
	am	pm			
	am	pm	/		
	am	pm			
	am	pm	/		
	am	pm			
	am	pm	/		
	am	pm			
	am	pm	/		
	am	pm			
	am	pm	/		
	am	pm			
	am	pm	/		
	am	pm			
	am	pm	/		
	am	pm			
	am	pm	/		
	am	pm			
	am	pm	/		
	am	pm			
	am	pm	/		
	am	pm			
	am	pm	/		

Blood Pressure Log

Date	Time		SYS/DIA [mmHg]	Pulse [Pul/min]	Notes
	am	pm			
	am	pm	/		
	am	pm			
	am	pm	/		
	am	pm			
	am	pm	/		
	am	pm			
	am	pm	/		
	am	pm			
	am	pm	/		
	am	pm			
	am	pm	/		
	am	pm			
	am	pm	/		
	am	pm			
	am	pm	/		
	am	pm			
	am	pm	/		
	am	pm			
	am	pm	/		
	am	pm			
	am	pm	/		
	am	pm			
	am	pm	/		

Blood Pressure Log

Date	Time am/pm	SYS/DIA [mmHg]	Pulse [Pul/min]	Notes
	am / pm	/		
	am / pm	/		
	am / pm	/		
	am / pm	/		
	am / pm	/		
	am / pm	/		
	am / pm	/		
	am / pm	/		
	am / pm	/		
	am / pm	/		
	am / pm	/		
	am / pm	/		

Blood Pressure Log

Date	Time		SYS/DIA [mmHg]	Pulse [Pul/min]	Notes
	am	pm			
	am	pm	/		....
	am	pm	/		....
	am	pm	/		....
	am	pm	/		....
	am	pm	/		....
	am	pm	/		....
	am	pm	/		....
	am	pm	/		....
	am	pm	/		....
	am	pm	/		....
	am	pm	/		....
	am	pm	/		....

Made in the USA
Las Vegas, NV
22 December 2024

15204545R00056